PALEO DIET

FRESH STARTERS

Ethan M. Sprouse

Contents

Contents

Chapter One

INTRODUCTION

The paleo diet is based on what our forefathers ate thousands of years ago as hunter-gatherers. Although it's impossible to say what our forefathers ate in different parts of the world, researchers believe their diets consisted of whole foods. Hunter-gatherers presumably had much lower rates of lifestyle diseases like obesity, diabetes, and heart disease because they ate a whole food-based diet and lived physically active lives. Several studies have found that following this diet can result in significant weight loss (without calorie counting) and significant health improvements. WHAT IS THE PALEO DIET AND WHY SHOULD YOU DO IT?

The Paleo Diet's central premise is straightforward: we should eat like people did before the Agricultural Revolution. Simple, unprocessed food that a hunter-gatherer would eat is the best food, according to this philosophy. The Paleo Diet is plant-centered, contrary to popular belief. It contains a lot of non-starchy vegetables (all the green, red, orange, and yellow ones), as well as some fruit in moderation. It contains meat, preferably unprocessed meat, and the more wild the better. Eggs, nuts and seeds, bugs, seafood, and fish are all included in this dish. There is a strong emphasis on eating seasonally and locally as much as possible, cooking your own food, and being physically active. Avoid processed foods, grains, legumes, and sugar, and instead drink mostly water, some tea or herbal infusions, and small amounts of fruit juice or alcohol on occasion. There is no one "right" way to eat for everyone, and paleolithic humans survived on a variety of diets based on what was available at the time and where they lived. Some people ate a low-carb, animal-based diet, while others ate a high-carb, plant-based diet. This should be regarded as a guideline rather than a rule of thumb. All of this can be customized to meet your specific requirements.

Chapter Two

THINGS TO STAY AWAY FROM

Soft drinks, fruit juices, table sugar, candy, pastries, ice cream, and numerous other products contain sugar and high-fructose corn syrup.

Wheat, spelt, rye, barley, and other grains are used in breads and pastas.

Beans, lentils, and a variety of other legumes are among the many types of legumes available.

Most dairy, especially low-fat dairy, should be avoided (some versions of paleo do include full-fat dairy like butter and cheese).

Soybean oil, sunflower oil, cottonseed oil, corn oil, grapeseed oil, safflower oil, and others are just a few examples of vegetable oils.

Margarine and a variety of processed foods contain trans fats. "Hydrogenated" or "partially hydrogenated" oils are the most common terms used to describe these oils.

Aspartame, sucralose, cyclamates, saccharin, and potassium acesulfame are examples of artificial sweeteners. Replace the sugar with natural sweeteners.

Everything labeled "diet" or "low-fat" or with a lot of additives is highly processed food. Artificial meal substitutes are included in this category.

A simple rule of thumb is to avoid eating anything that appears to have been manufactured.

Even on foods labeled as "health foods," ingredients lists must be read if you want to stay away from these ingredients.

EATING FOOD

Paleo foods should be the foundation of your diet:

Beef, lamb, chicken, turkey, pork, and a variety of other meats are all available.

Salmon, trout, haddock, shrimp, shellfish, and other varieties of fish and seafood are available. If you can, go for wild-caught.

Choose free-range, pastured, or omega-3-enhanced eggs when it comes to eggs.

Broccoli, kale, peppers, onions, carrots, tomatoes, and so on are some of the vegetables that can be used.

Apples, bananas, oranges, pears, avocados, strawberries, blueberries, and other fruits are among the fruits available.

Potatoes, sweet potatoes, yams, turnips, and other tubers are all examples of tubers.

Almonds, macadamia nuts, walnuts, hazelnuts, sunflower seeds, pumpkin seeds, and more are among the various nuts and seeds available.

Olive oil, avocado oil, and other healthy fats and oils

Sea salt, garlic, turmeric, rosemary, and other herbs and spices are examples of salt and spices.

If you can afford it, go for grass-fed, pasture-raised, and organic. If not, choose the least-processed option whenever possible. PALEO DIET RECIPES PERFECT BROKED SALMON

570 CAL/SERV CAL/SERV CAL/SERV CAL/SERV

SIZE OF YIELDS: 4 SIZE OF YIELDS: 4 SI

0 HOURS 10 MINUTES TO PREPARE

INGREDIENTS: 0 HOURS 20 MINS TOTAL TIME: 0 HOURS 20 MINS TOTAL TIME: 0 HOURS 20 MINS TOTAL TIME

Salmon fillets (4 oz.)

1 tablespoon mustard (grainy)

finely minced garlic cloves

a tablespoon of shallots, finely minced

1 teaspoon chopped fresh thyme leaves, plus more for garnish

a teaspoon of chopped fresh rosemary

lemon juice (half)

salt, kosher

Black pepper, freshly ground

For serving, lemon slices

DIRECTIONS

Preheat the oven to broil and prepare a parchment-lined baking sheet. Season with salt and pepper in a small mixing bowl with mustard, garlic, shallot, thyme, rosemary, and lemon juice. Broil for 7 to 8 minutes after spreading mixture over salmon fillets.

Serve garnished with additional thyme and lemon slices.

570 calories, 79 grams of protein, 1 gram of carbohydrates, 0 gram of fiber, 0 gram of sugar, 26 grams of fat, 4 grams of saturated fat, and 170 milligrams of sodium (per serving).

Paleo Chili Recipe of the Year

6 SERVINGS YIELDS

TIME TO PREPARE: 15 MINUTES 0 HOUR

INGREDIENTS: 0 HOURS 55 MINS TOTAL TIME: 0 HOURS 55 MINS TOTAL TIME: 0 HOURS 55 MINS TOTAL TIME

1/2-inch-thick slices of bacon

1/2 medium chopped yellow onion

2 sprigs celery (chopped)

chopped red and green peppers

garlic cloves, chopped

lean ground beef, 2 pound

chili powder (2 tbsp.)

2 tblsp cumin powder

2 tblsp oregano (dried)

smoked paprika (about 2 tbsp.)

salt, kosher

Black pepper, freshly ground

Fire-roasted tomatoes (28 oz.) from a can

c) chicken broth with low sodium

garnish with sliced jalapeos

Garnish with sliced avocado

cilantro, chopped

DIRECTIONS

Bacon should be cooked in a large pot on medium heat. Remove the bacon from the pot with a slotted spoon once it has become crispy. Cook for 6 minutes, or until onions, celery, and peppers are soft. Cook for another minute, until garlic is fragrant.

Remove the vegetables to one side of the pan and add the beef to the other. Cook until no pink remains, stirring occasionally. Return to the heat once the fat has been drained.

Season with salt and pepper after adding chili powder, cumin, oregano, and paprika. Cook for another 2 minutes, stirring occasionally. Bring to a simmer the tomatoes and broth. Cook for another 10 to 15 minutes, or until the chili has slightly thickened.

Place reserved bacon, jalapeos, cilantro, and avocado on top of the soup in bowls.

Paleo Meatloaf is a simple recipe that can be made in a matter of minutes.

6 SERVINGS YIELDS

TIME TO PREPARE: 15 MINUTES 0 HOUR

1 HOUR AND 15 MINUTES TOTAL

INGREDIENTS

spray for cooking

2 tbsp olive oil (extra virgin)

a finely chopped small onion

3 garlic cloves (chopped)

1 tsp oregano (dried)

salt, kosher

Black pepper, freshly ground

1 pound of beef (ground)

almond flour (half a cup)

2 oz.

2 tblsp coconut aminos (distributed)

Tomato paste (quarter cup)

apple cider vinegar, 2 tblsp.

garlic powder (1/2 teaspoon)

mustard powder (about 1/4 teaspoon)

1 tblsp. cayenne

DIRECTIONS

Preheat the oven to 350 degrees Fahrenheit (180 degrees Celsius). Use parchment paper to line a loaf pan and cooking spray to grease it. Heat the oil in a big skillet over medium heat. Cook for 5 minutes after adding the onion and garlic.

Salt and pepper to taste, along with oregano. Allow time for cooling.

Season beef, almond flour, eggs, 1 tablespoon coconut aminos, and onion mixture with salt and pepper in a big mixing bowl. Fill prepared pan with beef mixture.

Toss tomato paste, vinegar, 1 tablespoon coconut aminos, garlic powder, mustard powder, and cayenne pepper in a medium mixing bowl. Using salt and pepper, season to taste.

Coat the meatloaf in the mixture.

Bake for 1 hour, or until the meatloaf is fully cooked and the internal temperature reaches 155°. Remove from the pan and set aside for 15 minutes before serving. Paleo pizza perfection

4 SERVINGS YIELDS

0 HOURS 10 MINUTES TO PREPARE

TIME TOTAL: 30 MINUTES

INGREDIENTS

2 1/2 cups almond flour (plus a little extra for dusting)

baking powder (1/2 teaspoon)

1 teaspoon seasoning (Italian)

Garlic powder in a pinch

kosher salt (1/2 tsp.)

3 oz.

2 tbsp olive oil (extra virgin)

pizza sauce (1/2 cup)

c. mozzarella cheese (dairy-free)

pepperoni slices (about 1/4 cup)

1 thinly sliced small red onion

1/2 a thinly sliced small green bell pepper

black olives, sliced 1/4 cup

thickly sliced cremini mushrooms

1 tsp. crushed red pepper

DIRECTIONS

Preheat the oven to 425 degrees Fahrenheit and place a rack in the upper third of the oven. Mix almond flour, baking powder, Italian seasoning, garlic powder, and salt together in a large mixing bowl.

Whisk together the eggs and olive oil in a small bowl, then pour over the dry ingredients. To make a dough, combine all of the ingredients in a mixing bowl and stir until a Place dough on a parchment-lined baking sheet. Place a piece of parchment on top of the dough and roll it out to a thickness of 14 inches. Remove and discard the top sheet of parchment.

Place a baking sheet on top of the bottom parchment paper with the crust. Cook for about 10 minutes, or until the crust is lightly golden.

Make a 12-inch border around the pizza sauce on the crust. Return to the oven after topping with mozzarella and vegetable toppings. Bake for about 10 minutes, or until the cheese has melted and the crust is golden.

Preheat the oven to broil and cook for 2 minutes, or until the cheese is golden.

Prior to serving, sprinkle with red pepper flakes.

Baked Salmon in Garlic Butter

596 596 596 596 596 596 596 596 596 596 596 5

SIZE OF YIELDS: 4 SIZE OF YIELDS: 4 SI

0 HOURS 10 MINUTES TO PREPARE

INGREDIENTS: 0 HOURS 25 MINS TOTAL TIME: 0 HOURS 25 MINS TOTAL TIME: 0 HOURS 25 MINS TOTAL TIME

2 sliced lemons

1 fillet de saumon (about 3 lb.)

salt, kosher

Black pepper, freshly ground

melted butter (about 6 tbsp.)

honey (1 tbsp.)

garlic cloves, chopped

1 tbsp thyme leaves, chopped

1 tblsp oregano (dried)

Garnish with fresh chopped parsley

DIRECTIONS

Preheat the oven to 350 degrees Fahrenheit (180 degrees Celsius). Using foil and cooking spray, line a large rimmed baking sheet. Place lemon slices in an even layer across the foil's center.

Salt and pepper both sides of the salmon before placing it on top of the lemon slices.

Butter, honey, garlic, thyme, and oregano are whisked together in a small bowl. Pour the sauce over the salmon, then wrap it in foil. Cook for about 25 minutes, or until the salmon is fully cooked.

Preheat the oven to broil for 2 minutes, or until the butter mixture has thickened.

Before serving, top with parsley.

596 calories, 68 grams of protein, 11 grams of carbohydrates, 1 gram of fiber, 9 grams of sugar, 30 grams of fat, 14 grams of saturated fat, and 548 milligrams of sodium (per serving).

Paleo Bread to Die For

6 SERVINGS YIELDS

0 HOURS 10 MINUTES TO PREPARE

TIME TO COMPLETE: 0 HOURS 45 MINUTES TOTAL

INGREDIENTS

almond flour (about 2/3 cup)

flaxseed meal, 1 tablespoon

coconut flour (2 tbsp.)

baking soda, 2 tbsp.

kosher salt (1/2 tsp.)

5 oz.

extra-virgin olive oil (about a quarter cup)

agave syrup (1 tbsp.)

apple cider vinegar (1 tbsp.)

DIRECTIONS

Preheat the oven to 350°F and grease an 8"x5" loaf pan.

Almond flour, flaxseed meal, coconut flour, baking soda, and salt should all be combined in a large mixing bowl. Whisk together the eggs, olive oil, agave, and apple cider vinegar until smooth.

Using a spatula, smooth the top of the batter into the prepared loaf pan. Bake for 35 minutes, or until golden brown on top and a toothpick inserted in the center comes out clean. Before slicing, remove the loaf from the pan and cool completely. Cacciatore de 30 chickens

SIZE OF YIELDS: 4 SIZE OF YIELDS: 4 SI

0 HOURS 30 MINUTES TO PREPARE

TIME TOTAL: 30 MINUTES

INGREDIENTS

4 tbsp. fat de cuisine

1 pound chicken legs, bone-in and skin-on

chicken thighs (half a pound)

kosher salt (1/2 tsp.)

1 tblsp. black pepper, freshly ground

minced onion

finely chopped red bell pepper, 1/2

c. Slicing mushrooms

garlic cloves, chopped

1 tablespoon drained capers

1 tomato can (14.5 oz.) diced

1 c. water or chicken broth

1 tbsp. freshly chopped basil leaves

DIRECTIONS

2 tablespoons cooking fat, heated over medium-high heat and swirled to coat the bottom of a large skillet with high edges Salt and pepper the chicken before placing it in the pan. 3 minutes per side to sear the chicken until golden brown.

Set the chicken aside after removing it from the pan. Add the remaining 2 tablespoons cooking fat, onions, and peppers to the same pan on medium-high heat and cook for 2 to 3 minutes, or until the onion is translucent.

Cook, stirring for 2 minutes after adding the mushrooms. Stir in the garlic for about 1 minute, until fragrant, before adding the capers and diced tomatoes.

Return the chicken to the pan and add chicken broth or water to cover everything. Reduce the heat to medium-low and bring the mixture to a gentle simmer.

Reduce the heat to low and continue to cook (not boil) for another 30 minutes, or until the chicken reaches an internal temperature of 160°.

Burgers with lettuce, tomato, and bacon

980 980 980 980 980 980 980 980 980 980 980 9

SIZE OF YIELDS: 4 SIZE OF YIELDS: 4 SI

0 HOURS AND 25 MINUTES TO PREPARE

TOTAL TIME: 0 HUNDRED AND FIFTY-FIVE MINUTES

INGREDIENTS

halved 1 pound bacon slices

1 pound of beef (ground)

salt, kosher

black peppercorns, ground

mayonnaise (half a cup)

lemon juice (half)

3 tablespoons chives, finely chopped

Serve with butterhead lettuce.

slices of tomato

DIRECTIONS

Preheat the oven to 400 degrees and line a baking sheet with a baking rack (to help catch grease).

To make a bacon weave, place 3 bacon halves side by side on a baking rack. Place a fourth bacon half on top of the side pieces and beneath the middle slice by lifting one end of the middle bacon slice. Re-position the middle slice.

Lift the two side bacon strips and place a fifth bacon half on top of the middle piece and underneath the sides. Re-position the side slices.

Lift the other end of the middle slice and place a sixth slice on top of the side pieces and underneath the middle slice. Make a second weft by repeating the previous steps.

Season with salt and pepper, then bake for 25 minutes, or until the bacon is crisp. To blot grease, place on a plate lined with paper towels. Allow 10 minutes for cooling.

Prepare burgers in the meantime: Heat a grill (or a grill pan) to medium-high. Salt and pepper both sides of the ground beef patties. Grill for 4 minutes per side for medium.

Whisk together mayonnaise, lemon juice, and chives in a small bowl to make herb mayo.

Assemble the burgers: Place a bacon weave on the bottom of each burger and spread some herb mayo on top. Top with the remaining bacon weave, burger, lettuce, and tomato. Right away, serve.

980 calories, 67 grams of protein, 4 grams of carbohydrates, 1 gram of fiber, 2 grams of sugar, 75 grams of fat, 21 grams of saturated fat, and 2180 milligrams of sodium per serving

270 CAL/SERV CAL/SERV CAL/SERV CAL/SERV

SIZE OF YIELDS: 4 SIZE OF YIELDS: 4 SI

0 HOURS 10 MINUTES TO PREPARE

TIME TOTAL: ZERO HOURS AND TWENTY MINUTES

INGREDIENTS

a tablespoon of extra-virgin olive oil (divided)

steaks of swordfish

salt, kosher

Black pepper, freshly ground

a pound of halved multicolored cherry tomatoes

finely chopped 1/4 cup red onion

a tablespoon of basil, thinly sliced

DIRECTIONS FOR 1/2 LEMON JUICE

Preheat the oven to 400 degrees Fahrenheit (200 degrees Celsius).

2 tablespoons oil 2 tablespoons oil 2 tablespoons oil 2 tablespoons oil 2 tablespoons oil 2 tablespoons oil 2 tablespoons oil 2 tablespoons oil 2 tablespoons oil 2 tablespoons oil 2 tablespoons Season tops of fish with salt and pepper before adding to pan. 3 to 5 minutes until one side of the fish is browned. Season the other side with salt and pepper before flipping it over. Place the pan in the oven after it has been removed from the heat source.

Cook for 10 minutes, or until swordfish is flaky and cooked through.

To make the fresh tomato salad, toss tomatoes, onion, and basil in a large mixing bowl. Season with salt and pepper the remaining tablespoon of oil and the lemon juice.

Serve the fish with the salad on top.

270 calories, 21 grams of protein, 7 grams of carbohydrates, 2 grams of fiber, 4 grams of sugar, 18 grams of fat, 3 grams of saturated fat, and 90 milligrams of sodium (per serving).

Salmon with a Lemony Flavor on the Grill

SIZE OF YIELDS: 4 SIZE OF YIELDS: 4 SI

0 HOURS 10 MINUTES TO PREPARE

INGREDIENTS: 0 HOURS 20 MINS TOTAL TIME: 0 HOURS 20 MINS TOTAL TIME: 0 HOURS 20 MINS TOTAL TIME

Salmon fillets, 6 oz., skin-on

Brushing oil made from extra-virgin olives

salt, kosher

Black pepper, freshly ground

2 lemons, peeled and cut into wedges

butter, 2 tbsp.

DIRECTIONS

Heat grill to high. Brush salmon with oil and season with salt and pepper. Add salmon and lemon slices and grill until salmon is cooked through and lemons are charred, 5 minutes per side.

Add a pat of butter to salmon right when it's off the grill and top with grilled lemons. Serve. Sweet Potato Chili

6 SERVINGS YIELDS

TIME TO PREPARE: 15 MINUTES 0 HOUR

TOTAL TIME: 0 HOURS 50 MINS

INGREDIENTS

2 tbsp olive oil (extra virgin)

1 medium onion, chopped

1 bell pepper, chopped

3 garlic cloves (chopped)

1 tbsp. tomato paste

1 lb. Italian sausage

1 tbsp. chili powder

1 tblsp oregano (dried)

garlic powder (1/2 teaspoon)

1/4 tsp. cayenne

salt, kosher

Black pepper, freshly ground

4 large sweet potatoes, peeled and cubed into 1" pieces

3 c. low-sodium chicken broth

1 (14.5-oz.) can diced tomatoes

Freshly chopped parsley, for serving

DIRECTIONS

In a large pot over medium heat, heat oil. Add onion and bell pepper and cook until soft, 5 minutes. Add garlic and cook until fragrant, 1 minute more, then add tomato paste and stir until well coated. Add sausage and cook, breaking up meat with a wooden spoon until no longer pink, 7 minutes. Add chili powder, oregano, garlic powder, and cayenne and season with salt and pepper.

Add sweet potatoes, broth, and tomatoes and bring to a boil. Reduce heat and let simmer, covered, until sweet potatoes are tender, about 15 minutes.

Before serving, top with parsley.

Slow-Cooker Paleo Meatballs

YIELDS: 24

TIME TO PREPARE: 15 MINUTES 0 HOUR

TOTAL TIME: 5 HOURS 45 MINS

INGREDIENTS

FOR MEATBALLS

1 1/2 lb. ground beef

1/4 c. freshly chopped parsley, plus more for garnish

large egg

garlic cloves, minced 1 tsp.

salt, kosher

1/2 tsp. crushed red pepper flakes

FOR SAUCE

1 (28-oz.) can crushed tomatoes

(6-oz.) can tomato paste

1/4 yellow onion, finely chopped

1 tsp oregano (dried)

1 garlic clove, minced

salt, kosher

Black pepper, freshly ground

DIRECTIONS

Make meatballs: In a large bowl, mix together beef, parsley, egg, garlic, salt, and red pepper flakes until combined. Form mixture into 24 meatballs and place in slow cooker.

Make sauce: In another large bowl, stir together crushed tomatoes, tomato paste, onion, oregano, and garlic and season with salt and pepper. Pour over meatballs.

Cook, covered, on low until meatballs are cooked through, 5 to 5 1/2 hours.

Before serving, top with parsley.

Paleo Breakfast Stacks

YIELDS: 3 SERVINGS

0 HOURS 10 MINUTES TO PREPARE

TIME TOTAL: 30 MINUTES

INGREDIENTS

3 breakfast sausage patties

1 avocado, mashed

salt, kosher

Black pepper, freshly ground

3 oz.

chives, for garnish

Hot sauce, if desired

DIRECTIONS

Heat breakfast sausage according to instructions on box.

Mash avocado onto breakfast sausage and season with salt and pepper.

Spray a medium skillet over medium heat with cooking spray, then spray the inside of a mason jar lid. Place mason jar lid in center of skillet and crack an egg inside. Season with salt and pepper and let cook 3 minutes until whites are set, then remove lid and continue cooking.

Place egg on top of mashed avocado. Garnish with chives and drizzle with your favorite hot sauce. Paleo Banana Bread

6 SERVINGS YIELDS

TIME TO PREPARE: 15 MINUTES 0 HOUR

TOTAL TIME: 1 HOUR 0 MINS

INGREDIENTS

1/3 c. coconut flour

1/4 c. almond flour

1/2 tsp. ground cinnamon

baking powder (1/2 teaspoon)

1/2 tsp. baking soda

kosher salt (1/2 tsp.)

1/4 c. coconut oil

1/4 c. smooth unsweetened almond butter

2 large ripe bananas, mashed (about 1 c.)

2 tbsp. agave syrup

tbsp. pure vanilla extract

large eggs

DIRECTIONS

Preheat oven to 350° and line an 8"-x-5" loaf pan with parchment paper. In a medium bowl, whisk to combine coconut flour, almond flour, cinnamon, baking powder, baking soda, and salt.

In a large, microwave-safe bowl, combine coconut oil and almond butter. Microwave until coconut oil is melted and almond butter is more liquid, 10 seconds on high. Whisk in mashed bananas, agave, and vanilla, then whisk in eggs. Gently fold in dry ingredients until just combined.

Pour batter into prepared pan and bake 40 to 45 minutes, until top is golden and a toothpick inserted into the center comes out clean. Let cool completely before slicing. Bell Pepper Eggs

YIELDS: 3

PREP TIME: 0 HOURS 5 MINS

TIME TOTAL: ZERO HOURS AND TWENTY MINUTES

INGREDIENTS

1 bell pepper, sliced into 1/4" rings

6 eggs

salt, kosher

Freshly ground black peppers

2 tbsp. Chopped chives

2 tbsp. chopped parsley

DIRECTIONS

Heat a nonstick skillet over medium heat, and grease lightly with cooking spray.

Place a bell pepper ring in the skillet, then sauté for two minutes. Flip the ring, then crack an egg in the middle. Season with salt and pepper, then cook until the egg is cooked to your liking, 2 to 4 minutes. Repeat with the other eggs, then garnish with chives and parsley. One-Pan Balsamic Chicken and Asparagus

SIZE OF YIELDS: 4 SIZE OF YIELDS: 4 SI

PREP TIME: 0 HOURS 20 MINS

TIME TOTAL: ZERO HOURS AND TWENTY MINUTES

INGREDIENTS

1/4 c. balsamic vinegar

1/4 c. extra-virgin olive oil, divided

1 tbsp. honey

tbsp. Dijon mustard

garlic cloves, chopped

pinch of crushed red pepper flakes

2 lb. chicken breast tenders

salt, kosher

Black pepper, freshly ground

1 lb. asparagus, woody ends trimmed

1 pt. cherry tomatoes, halved

DIRECTIONS

Make vinaigrette: In a small bowl, whisk together balsamic, 2 tablespoons oil, honey, mustard, garlic, and red pepper flakes until combined. Set aside.

In a large skillet over medium heat, heat remaining oil. Add chicken, season with salt and pepper, and sear until golden, about 3 minutes per side. Remove from pan and set aside.

To pan, add asparagus and tomatoes, season with more salt and pepper, and cook until asparagus is bright green and tomatoes are slightly wilted, 5 minutes or so.

Move veggies to one side, add chicken back in and pour in vinaigrette. Toss veggies and chicken slightly until chicken is cooked through and vinaigrette is thickened, 5 minutes more. Broccoli Salad

YIELDS: 4 - 6 SERVINGS

PREP TIME: 0 HOURS 20 MINS

TOTAL TIME: 0 HUNDRED AND FIFTY-FIVE MINUTES

INGREDIENTS

FOR THE SALAD

salt, kosher

3 heads broccoli, cut into bite-size pieces

2 carrots, shredded

1/2 red onion, thinly sliced

1/2 c. dried cranberries

1/2 c. sliced almonds

6 slices bacon, cooked and crumbled

FOR THE DRESSING

mayonnaise (half a cup)

3 tbsp. apple cider vinegar

salt, kosher

Black pepper, freshly ground

DIRECTIONS

In a medium sauce pan, bring 4 cups of salted water to a boil. While waiting for the water to boil, prepare a large bowl with ice water.

Add broccoli florets to the boiling water and cook until tender, 1 to 2 minutes. Remove with a slotted spoon and place in the prepared bowl of ice water. When cool, drain florets in a colander.

In a large bowl, combine broccoli, carrots, red onion, cranberries, almonds and bacon.

In a medium bowl, whisk together mayonnaise and vinegar and season with salt and pepper.

Pour dressing over broccoli mixture and stir to combine.

Classic Chicken Salad

YIELDS: 8 - 10

0 HOURS 10 MINUTES TO PREPARE

TIME TOTAL: ZERO HOURS AND TWENTY MINUTES

INGREDIENTS

3 chicken breasts

green apple, chopped

1/2 red onion, finely chopped

celery stalks, finely chopped

2/3 c. mayonnaise

2 tbsp. lemon juice

salt, kosher

Freshly cracked black pepper

1 tbsp. chopped dill, for garnish

6 slices lemon (optional)

6 sprigs dill (optional)

DIRECTIONS

Poach chicken: In a large pot, arrange the chicken breasts in a single layer. If using, place lemon slices and dill sprigs on chicken. Pour water over the chicken breasts, covering by at least an inch. Bring water to a boil, then reduce to simmer and cook for 10 minutes or until the center of the chicken reaches 165° with an instant read thermometer. If you don't have a thermometer, check that the thickest part of the chicken is opaque.

Slice chicken into bite-sized pieces.

In a large bowl, combine chicken, apple, onion and celery.

In a medium bowl, combine mayonnaise and lemon juice and season with salt and pepper. Whisk until combined.

Pour dressing over chicken mixture and toss. Garnish with dill and serve. Tuna Salad Pickle Boats

YIELDS: 6

TIME TO PREPARE: 15 MINUTES 0 HOUR

TOTAL TIME: 0 HOURS 15 MINS

INGREDIENTS

2 5-oz. cans tuna, drained

1/4 c. mayonnaise

tbsp. Dijon mustard

stalks celery, finely chopped

Juice of 1/2 a lemon

1 tbsp. chopped dill, plus more for garnish

salt, kosher

Black pepper, freshly ground

6 dill pickles

Paprika, for garnish

DIRECTIONS

In a large bowl, combine tuna, mayo, Dijon, celery, lemon juice, and dill. Mix until combined and season with salt and pepper.

Slice pickles in half lengthwise. Using a spoon, scoop out the seeds to create boats. Fill boats with tuna salad and garnish with paprika and more dill Breakfast Tomatoes

YIELDS: 3

PREP TIME: 0 HOURS 5 MINS

TIME TO COMPLETE: 0 HOURS 45 MINUTES TOTAL

INGREDIENTS

3 large tomatoes

1 tbsp. olive oil

salt, kosher

Black pepper, freshly ground

3 eggs

1 tbsp. chives, thinly chopped

freshly grated Parmesan, for serving

DIRECTIONS

Preheat oven to 400° and line a small baking sheet with parchment paper. Slice tops off tomatoes and hollow with a metal spoon. Drizzle with olive oil and season with salt and pepper. Place in oven and bake 10 minutes, until softened slightly. Crack eggs into center and place back in oven to bake 12 to 15 minutes more, until egg is cooked to your preference. Season with more salt and pepper and garnish with chives and parmesan. Serve. Brussels Sprouts Hash

4 SERVINGS YIELDS

0 HOURS 10 MINUTES TO PREPARE

TOTAL TIME: 0 HOURS 40 MINS

INGREDIENTS

6 slices bacon, cut into 1" pieces

1/2 onion, chopped

lb. Brussels sprouts, trimmed and quartered

salt, kosher

Black pepper, freshly ground

1/4 tsp. crushed red pepper flakes

garlic cloves, chopped

4 large eggs

DIRECTIONS

In a large skillet over medium heat, cook bacon until crispy. Turn off heat and transfer bacon to a paper towel-lined plate. Drain all but about 1 tablespoon bacon fat.

Turn heat back to medium and add onion and Brussels sprouts to the skillet. Cook, stirring occasionally, until vegetables begin to soften and turn golden. Season with salt, pepper, and red pepper flakes.

Add 2 tablespoons of water and cover skillet. Cook until Brussels sprouts are tender and water has evaporated, about 5 minutes. (If all the water evaporates before the Brussels sprouts are tender, add more water to skillet and cover for a couple minutes more.) Add garlic to skillet and cook until fragrant, 1 minute.

Using a wooden spoon, make four holes in the hash to reveal bottom of skillet. Crack an egg into each hole and season each egg with salt and pepper. Replace lid and cook until eggs are cooked to your liking, about 5 minutes for a just runny egg.

Sprinkle cooked bacon bits over entire skillet and serve warm

Grilled Chicken

4 SERVINGS YIELDS

TIME TO PREPARE: 15 MINUTES 0 HOUR

TIME TO COMPLETE: 0 HOURS 45 MINUTES TOTAL

INGREDIENTS

1/4 c. balsamic vinegar

3 tbsp.extra-virgin olive oil

tbsp. brown sugar

garlic cloves, chopped

1 tsp. dried thyme

1 tsp. dried rosemary

4 chicken breasts

salt, kosher

Black pepper, freshly ground

Freshly chopped parsley, for garnish

DIRECTIONS

In a medium bowl, whisk together balsamic vinegar, olive oil, brown sugar, garlic, and dried herbs, and season generously with salt and pepper. Reserve ¼ cup.

Add chicken to the bowl and toss to combine. Let marinate at least 20 minutes and up to overnight.

Preheat grill to medium high. Add chicken and grill, basting with reserved marinade, until cooked through, 6 minutes per side.

Before serving, top with parsley.

Paleo Chocolate Chip Cookies

YIELDS:

0 HOURS 10 MINUTES TO PREPARE

TOTAL TIME: 0 HOURS 25 MINS

INGREDIENTS

c. almond flour

1/2 tsp. baking soda

1/4 tsp. kosher salt

1/4 c. butter, room temperature

1/4 c. almond butter

honey (1 tbsp.)

1 large egg

1 tsp. pure vanilla extract

1 c. semisweet chocolate chips

Flaky sea salt

DIRECTIONS

Preheat oven to 350° and line a baking sheet with parchment paper. In a large bowl, whisk together almond flour, baking soda, and salt. Add butter, almond butter, honey, egg, and vanilla and, using a hand mixer, beat until combined.

Fold in chocolate chips until combined, then add tablespoonfuls of batter to prepared baking sheet. Sprinkle cookies with flaky sea salt.

Bake until edges are golden, 13 to 15 minutes.

Balsamic Grilled Chicken and Zucchini

SIZE OF YIELDS: 4 SIZE OF YIELDS: 4 SI

0 HOURS 10 MINUTES TO PREPARE

TOTAL TIME: 0 HUNDRED AND FIFTY-FIVE MINUTES

INGREDIENTS

1/2 c. honey

1/2 c. balsamic vinegar

1 tbsp. orange zest

tsp. chopped fresh oregano

medium yellow zucchini (about 1 lb.)

2 medium green zucchini (about 1 lb.)

salt, kosher

1 1/2 lb. Tyson Boneless Skinless Chicken Breasts, pounded to 1/2" thickness

extra-virgin olive oil

Chapter Three

Black pepper, freshly ground

DIRECTIONS

In a small sauce pan over medium heat add honey and balsamic vinegar. Bring to a boil and simmer until slightly thickened, 10 minutes. Turn off heat; stir in orange zest and oregano. Reserve 1/4 cup for serving.

Meanwhile, trim off both ends of each zucchini. Using a mandoline or vegetable peeler, create long flat noodles by running the blade against the length of each zucchini. Season with salt and set aside.

Preheat grill on medium-high. Drizzle Tyson Boneless Skinless Chicken Breastswith olive oil and season with salt and pepper. Place chicken on grill and cook for 4 minutes on each side. Brush glaze onto chicken and cook until lightly charred all over and internal temperature reaches 170°, 2 to 3 minutes. Transfer to a clean plate and cover loosely with foil.

Bring an 8-quart stock pot of water to a boil and generously season with salt. Cook zucchini until al dente, 2 to 3 minutes, and drain. Slice chicken against the grain and serve over zucchini noodles with a drizzle of balsamic-honey glaze and a sprinkle of sea salt. Right away, serve. Parmesan-Crusted Salmon

4 SERVINGS YIELDS

PREP TIME: 0 HOURS 5 MINS

TIME TOTAL: ZERO HOURS AND TWENTY MINUTES

INGREDIENTS

1 c. grated Parmesan, plus more for garnish

1/4 c. chopped parsley, plus more for garnish

1 tblsp oregano (dried)

4 salmon pieces, about 2 lbs.

extra-virgin olive oil

salt, kosher

Black pepper, freshly ground

1 head broccoli, cut into florets

DIRECTIONS

In a small bowl combine parmesan, parsley and oregano. Rub salmon with olive oil and season with salt and black pepper. Place handful of cheese mixture on top of each piece; press down lightly to adhere.

Preheat oven to 425 degrees F. In a large cast iron skillet or nonstick pan over medium heat carefully place 2 pieces of salmon cheese-side down and sear until golden; about 2 to 3 minutes. Transfer to a plate cheese-side up. Wipe pan to remove excess cheese and repeat with remaining salmon. Place all salmon cheese-side up in the skillet and bake until cooked through, about 4 minutes.

Meanwhile, bring a large pot filled with salted water to a boil and cook broccoli for 2 minutes.

Plate salmon and drizzle with olive oil; garnish with parsley and parmesan. Serve immediately with broccoli. HEALTH BENEFITS OF PALEO DIET

Promotes healthy blood glucose

Improved insulin sensitivity

Lower blood pressure

Weight management including reduced waist circumference

Improved cholesterol balance

Improved satiety

Lower all-cause mortality

CONCLUSION

Our modern food is heavily processed, reliant on grains and sugars and modified fats. Most of the chronic health concerns that plague Americans today weren't as problematic in the past. The Paleo Diet posits that our food may be contributing to these diseases. As with any significant dietary change, it is best to consult your doctor before diving into the Paleo Diet. If you have the desire and time to prepare your own food and to get physically active, then a Paleolithic-type diet may work for you. Remember it is always important to work with your doctor and to pay attention to how your body responds.INGREDIENTS

6 slices bacon, cut into 1" pieces

1/2 onion, chopped

lb. Brussels sprouts, trimmed and quartered

salt, kosher

Black pepper, freshly ground

1/4 tsp. crushed red pepper flakes

garlic cloves, chopped

4 large eggs

DIRECTIONS

In a large skillet over medium heat, cook bacon until crispy. Turn off heat and transfer bacon to a paper towel-lined plate. Drain all but about 1 tablespoon bacon fat.

Turn heat back to medium and add onion and Brussels sprouts to the skillet. Cook, stirring occasionally, until vegetables begin to soften and turn golden. Season with salt, pepper, and red pepper flakes.

Add 2 tablespoons of water and cover skillet. Cook until Brussels sprouts are tender and water has evaporated, about 5 minutes. (If all the water evaporates before the Brussels sprouts are tender, add more water to skillet and cover for a couple minutes more.) Add garlic to skillet and cook until fragrant, 1 minute.

Using a wooden spoon, make four holes in the hash to reveal bottom of skillet. Crack an egg into each hole and season each egg with salt and pepper. Replace lid and cook until eggs are cooked to your liking, about 5 minutes for a just runny egg.

Sprinkle cooked bacon bits over entire skillet and serve warm

Grilled Chicken

4 SERVINGS YIELDS

TIME TO PREPARE: 15 MINUTES 0 HOUR

TIME TO COMPLETE: 0 HOURS 45 MINUTES TOTAL

INGREDIENTS

1/4 c. balsamic vinegar

3 tbsp.extra-virgin olive oil

tbsp. brown sugar

garlic cloves, chopped

1 tsp. dried thyme

1 tsp. dried rosemary

4 chicken breasts

salt, kosher

Black pepper, freshly ground

Freshly chopped parsley, for garnish

DIRECTIONS

In a medium bowl, whisk together balsamic vinegar, olive oil, brown sugar, garlic, and dried herbs, and season generously with salt and pepper. Reserve ¼ cup.

Add chicken to the bowl and toss to combine. Let marinate at least 20 minutes and up to overnight.

Preheat grill to medium high. Add chicken and grill, basting with reserved marinade, until cooked through, 6 minutes per side.

Before serving, top with parsley.

Paleo Chocolate Chip Cookies

YIELDS:

0 HOURS 10 MINUTES TO PREPARE

TOTAL TIME: 0 HOURS 25 MINS

INGREDIENTS

c. almond flour

1/2 tsp. baking soda

1/4 tsp. kosher salt

1/4 c. butter, room temperature

1/4 c. almond butter

honey (1 tbsp.)

1 large egg

1 tsp. pure vanilla extract

1 c. semisweet chocolate chips

Flaky sea salt

DIRECTIONS

Preheat oven to 350° and line a baking sheet with parchment paper. In a large bowl, whisk together almond flour, baking soda, and salt. Add butter, almond butter, honey, egg, and vanilla and, using a hand mixer, beat until combined.

Fold in chocolate chips until combined, then add tablespoonfuls of batter to prepared baking sheet. Sprinkle cookies with flaky sea salt.

Bake until edges are golden, 13 to 15 minutes.

Balsamic Grilled Chicken and Zucchini

SIZE OF YIELDS: 4 SIZE OF YIELDS: 4 SI

0 HOURS 10 MINUTES TO PREPARE

TOTAL TIME: 0 HUNDRED AND FIFTY-FIVE MINUTES

INGREDIENTS

1/2 c. honey

1/2 c. balsamic vinegar

1 tbsp. orange zest

tsp. chopped fresh oregano

medium yellow zucchini (about 1 lb.)

2 medium green zucchini (about 1 lb.)

salt, kosher

1 1/2 lb. Tyson Boneless Skinless Chicken Breasts, pounded to 1/2" thickness

extra-virgin olive oil

Black pepper, freshly ground

sea salt, such as Maldon

DIRECTIONS

In a small sauce pan over medium heat add honey and balsamic vinegar. Bring to a boil and simmer until slightly thickened, 10 minutes. Turn off heat; stir in orange zest and oregano. Reserve 1/4 cup for serving.

Meanwhile, trim off both ends of each zucchini. Using a mandoline or vegetable peeler, create long flat noodles by running the blade against the length of each zucchini. Season with salt and set aside.

Preheat grill on medium-high. Drizzle Tyson Boneless Skinless Chicken Breastswith olive oil and season with salt and pepper. Place chicken on grill and cook for 4 minutes on each side. Brush glaze onto chicken and cook until lightly charred all over and internal temperature reaches 170°, 2 to 3 minutes. Transfer to a clean plate and cover loosely with foil.

Bring an 8-quart stock pot of water to a boil and generously season with salt. Cook zucchini until al dente, 2 to 3 minutes, and drain. Slice chicken against the grain and serve over zucchini noodles with a drizzle of balsamic-honey glaze and a sprinkle of sea salt. Right away, serve. Parmesan-Crusted Salmon

4 SERVINGS YIELDS

PREP TIME: 0 HOURS 5 MINS

TIME TOTAL: ZERO HOURS AND TWENTY MINUTES

INGREDIENTS

1 c. grated Parmesan, plus more for garnish

1/4 c. chopped parsley, plus more for garnish

1 tblsp oregano (dried)

4 salmon pieces, about 2 lbs.

extra-virgin olive oil

salt, kosher

Black pepper, freshly ground

1 head broccoli, cut into florets

DIRECTIONS

In a small bowl combine parmesan, parsley and oregano. Rub salmon with olive oil and season

with salt and black pepper. Place handful of cheese mixture on top of each piece; press down lightly to adhere.

Preheat oven to 425 degrees F. In a large cast iron skillet or nonstick pan over medium heat carefully place 2 pieces of salmon cheese-side down and sear until golden; about 2 to 3 minutes. Transfer to a plate cheese-side up. Wipe pan to remove excess cheese and repeat with remaining salmon.

Place all salmon cheese-side up in the skillet and bake until cooked through, about 4 minutes.

Meanwhile, bring a large pot filled with salted water to a boil and cook broccoli for 2 minutes.

Plate salmon and drizzle with olive oil; garnish with parsley and parmesan. Serve immediately with broccoli. HEALTH BENEFITS OF PALEO DIET

Promotes healthy blood glucose

Improved insulin sensitivity

Lower blood pressure

Weight management including reduced waist circumference

Improved cholesterol balance

Improved satiety

Lower all-cause mortality

CONCLUSION

Our modern food is heavily processed, reliant on grains and sugars and modified fats. Most of the chronic health concerns that plague Americans today weren't as problematic in the past. The Paleo Diet posits that our food may be contributing to these diseases. As with any significant dietary change, it is best to consult your doctor before diving into the Paleo Diet. If you have the desire and time to prepare your own food and to get physically active, then a Paleolithic-type diet may work for you. Remember it is always important to work with your doctor and to pay attention to how your body responds.INGREDIENTS

6 slices bacon, cut into 1" pieces

1/2 onion, chopped

lb. Brussels sprouts, trimmed and quartered

salt, kosher

Black pepper, freshly ground

1/4 tsp. crushed red pepper flakes

garlic cloves, chopped

4 large eggs

DIRECTIONS

In a large skillet over medium heat, cook bacon until crispy. Turn off heat and transfer bacon to a paper towel-lined plate. Drain all but about 1 tablespoon bacon fat.

Turn heat back to medium and add onion and Brussels sprouts to the skillet. Cook, stirring occasionally, until vegetables begin to soften and turn golden. Season with salt, pepper, and red pepper flakes.

Add 2 tablespoons of water and cover skillet. Cook until Brussels sprouts are tender and water has evaporated, about

5 minutes. (If all the water evaporates before the Brussels sprouts are tender, add more water to skillet and cover for a couple minutes more.) Add garlic to skillet and cook until fragrant, 1 minute.

Using a wooden spoon, make four holes in the hash to reveal bottom of skillet. Crack an egg into each hole and season each egg with salt and pepper. Replace lid and cook until eggs are cooked to your liking, about 5 minutes for a just runny egg.

Sprinkle cooked bacon bits over entire skillet and serve warm

Grilled Chicken

4 SERVINGS YIELDS

TIME TO PREPARE: 15 MINUTES 0 HOUR

TIME TO COMPLETE: 0 HOURS 45 MINUTES TOTAL

INGREDIENTS

1/4 c. balsamic vinegar

3 tbsp.extra-virgin olive oil

tbsp. brown sugar

garlic cloves, chopped

1 tsp. dried thyme

1 tsp. dried rosemary

4 chicken breasts

salt, kosher

Black pepper, freshly ground

Freshly chopped parsley, for garnish

DIRECTIONS

In a medium bowl, whisk together balsamic vinegar, olive oil, brown sugar, garlic, and dried herbs, and season generously with salt and pepper. Reserve ¼ cup.

Add chicken to the bowl and toss to combine. Let marinate at least 20 minutes and up to overnight.

Preheat grill to medium high. Add chicken and grill, basting with reserved marinade, until cooked through, 6 minutes per side.

Before serving, top with parsley.

Paleo Chocolate Chip Cookies

YIELDS:

0 HOURS 10 MINUTES TO PREPARE

TOTAL TIME: 0 HOURS 25 MINS

INGREDIENTS

c. almond flour

1/2 tsp. baking soda

1/4 tsp. kosher salt

1/4 c. butter, room temperature

1/4 c. almond butter

honey (1 tbsp.)

1 large egg

1 tsp. pure vanilla extract

1 c. semisweet chocolate chips

Flaky sea salt

DIRECTIONS

Preheat oven to 350° and line a baking sheet with parchment paper. In a large bowl, whisk together almond flour, baking soda, and salt. Add butter, almond butter, honey, egg, and vanilla and, using a hand mixer, beat until combined.

Fold in chocolate chips until combined, then add tablespoonfuls of batter to prepared baking sheet. Sprinkle cookies with flaky sea salt.

Bake until edges are golden, 13 to 15 minutes.

Balsamic Grilled Chicken and Zucchini

SIZE OF YIELDS: 4 SIZE OF YIELDS: 4 SI

0 HOURS 10 MINUTES TO PREPARE

TOTAL TIME: 0 HUNDRED AND FIFTY-FIVE MINUTES

INGREDIENTS

1/2 c. honey

1/2 c. balsamic vinegar

1 tbsp. orange zest

tsp. chopped fresh oregano

medium yellow zucchini (about 1 lb.)

2 medium green zucchini (about 1 lb.)

salt, kosher

1 1/2 lb. Tyson Boneless Skinless Chicken Breasts, pounded to 1/2" thickness

extra-virgin olive oil

Black pepper, freshly ground

sea salt, such as Maldon

DIRECTIONS

In a small sauce pan over medium heat add honey and balsamic vinegar. Bring to a boil and simmer until slightly thickened, 10 minutes. Turn off heat; stir in orange zest and oregano. Reserve 1/4 cup for serving.

Meanwhile, trim off both ends of each zucchini. Using a mandoline or vegetable peeler, create long flat noodles by running the blade against the length of each zucchini. Season with salt and set aside.

Preheat grill on medium-high. Drizzle Tyson Boneless Skinless Chicken Breastswith olive oil and season with salt and pepper. Place chicken on grill and cook for 4 minutes on each side. Brush glaze onto chicken and cook until lightly charred all over and internal temperature reaches 170°, 2 to 3 minutes. Transfer to a clean plate and cover loosely with foil.

Bring an 8-quart stock pot of water to a boil and generously season with salt. Cook zucchini until al dente, 2 to 3 minutes, and drain. Slice chicken against the grain and serve over zucchini noodles with a drizzle of balsamic-honey glaze and a sprinkle of sea salt. Right away, serve. Parmesan-Crusted Salmon

4 SERVINGS YIELDS

PREP TIME: 0 HOURS 5 MINS

TIME TOTAL: ZERO HOURS AND TWENTY MINUTES

INGREDIENTS

1 c. grated Parmesan, plus more for garnish

1/4 c. chopped parsley, plus more for garnish

1 tblsp oregano (dried)

4 salmon pieces, about 2 lbs.

extra-virgin olive oil

salt, kosher

Black pepper, freshly ground

1 head broccoli, cut into florets

DIRECTIONS

In a small bowl combine parmesan, parsley and oregano. Rub salmon with olive oil and season

with salt and black pepper. Place handful of cheese mixture on top of each piece; press down lightly to adhere.

Preheat oven to 425 degrees F. In a large cast iron skillet or nonstick pan over medium heat carefully place 2 pieces of salmon cheese-side down and sear until golden; about 2 to 3 minutes. Transfer to a plate cheese-side up. Wipe pan to remove excess cheese and repeat with remaining salmon. Place all salmon cheese-side up in the skillet and bake until cooked through, about 4 minutes.

Meanwhile, bring a large pot filled with salted water to a boil and cook broccoli for 2 minutes.

Plate salmon and drizzle with olive oil; garnish with parsley and parmesan. Serve immediately with broccoli. HEALTH BENEFITS OF PALEO DIET

Promotes healthy blood glucose

Improved insulin sensitivity

Lower blood pressure

Weight management including reduced waist circumference

Improved cholesterol balance

Improved satiety

Lower all-cause mortality

Chapter Four

Rub salmon with olive oil and season

In a small bowl combine parmesan, parsley and oregano.

with salt and black pepper. Place handful of cheese mixture on top of each piece; press down lightly to adhere.

Preheat oven to 425 degrees F. In a large cast iron skillet or nonstick pan over medium heat carefully place 2 pieces of salmon cheese-side down and sear until golden; about 2 to 3 minutes. Transfer to a plate cheese-side up. Wipe pan to remove excess cheese and repeat with remaining salmon. Place all salmon cheese-side up in the skillet and bake until cooked through, about 4 minutes.

Meanwhile, bring a large pot filled with salted water to a boil and cook broccoli for 2 minutes.

Plate salmon and drizzle with olive oil; garnish with parsley and parmesan. Serve immediately with broccoli. HEALTH BENEFITS OF PALEO DIET

Promotes healthy blood glucose

Improved insulin sensitivity

Lower blood pressure

Weight management including reduced waist circumference

Improved cholesterol balance

Improved satiety

Lower all-cause mortality

CONCLUSION

Our modern food is heavily processed, reliant on grains and sugars and modified fats. Most of the chronic health concerns that plague Americans today weren't as problematic in the past. The Paleo Diet posits that our food may be contributing to these diseases. As with any significant dietary change, it is best to consult your doctor before diving into the Paleo Diet. If you have the desire and time to prepare your own food and to get physically active, then a Paleolithic-type diet may work for you. Remember it is always important to work with your doctor and to pay attention to how your body responds.INGREDIENTS

6 slices bacon, cut into 1" pieces

1/2 onion, chopped

lb. Brussels sprouts, trimmed and quartered

salt, kosher

Black pepper, freshly ground

1/4 tsp. crushed red pepper flakes

garlic cloves, chopped

4 large eggs

DIRECTIONS

In a large skillet over medium heat, cook bacon until crispy. Turn off heat and transfer bacon to a paper towel-lined plate. Drain all but about 1 tablespoon bacon fat.

Turn heat back to medium and add onion and Brussels sprouts to the skillet. Cook, stirring occasionally, until vegetables begin to soften and turn golden. Season with salt, pepper, and red pepper flakes.

Add 2 tablespoons of water and cover skillet. Cook until Brussels sprouts are tender and water has evaporated, about 5 minutes. (If all the water evaporates before the Brussels sprouts are tender, add more water to skillet and cover for a couple minutes more.) Add garlic to skillet and cook until fragrant, 1 minute.

Using a wooden spoon, make four holes in the hash to reveal bottom of skillet. Crack an egg into each hole and season each egg with salt and pepper. Replace lid and cook until eggs are cooked to your liking, about 5 minutes for a just runny egg.

Sprinkle cooked bacon bits over entire skillet and serve warm

Grilled Chicken

4 SERVINGS YIELDS

TIME TO PREPARE: 15 MINUTES 0 HOUR

TIME TO COMPLETE: 0 HOURS 45 MINUTES TOTAL

INGREDIENTS

1/4 c. balsamic vinegar

3 tbsp.extra-virgin olive oil

tbsp. brown sugar

garlic cloves, chopped

1 tsp. dried thyme

1 tsp. dried rosemary

4 chicken breasts

salt, kosher

Black pepper, freshly ground

Freshly chopped parsley, for garnish

DIRECTIONS

In a medium bowl, whisk together balsamic vinegar, olive oil, brown sugar, garlic, and dried herbs, and season generously with salt and pepper. Reserve ¼ cup.

Add chicken to the bowl and toss to combine. Let marinate at least 20 minutes and up to overnight.

Preheat grill to medium high. Add chicken and grill, basting with reserved marinade, until cooked through, 6 minutes per side.

Before serving, top with parsley.

Paleo Chocolate Chip Cookies

YIELDS:

0 HOURS 10 MINUTES TO PREPARE

TOTAL TIME: 0 HOURS 25 MINS

INGREDIENTS

c. almond flour

1/2 tsp. baking soda

1/4 tsp. kosher salt

1/4 c. butter, room temperature

1/4 c. almond butter

honey (1 tbsp.)

1 large egg

1 tsp. pure vanilla extract

1 c. semisweet chocolate chips

Flaky sea salt

DIRECTIONS

Preheat oven to 350° and line a baking sheet with parchment paper. In a large bowl, whisk together almond flour, baking soda, and salt. Add butter, almond butter, honey, egg, and vanilla and, using a hand mixer, beat until combined.

Fold in chocolate chips until combined, then add tablespoonfuls of batter to prepared baking sheet. Sprinkle cookies with flaky sea salt.

Bake until edges are golden, 13 to 15 minutes.

Balsamic Grilled Chicken and Zucchini

SIZE OF YIELDS: 4 SIZE OF YIELDS: 4 SI

0 HOURS 10 MINUTES TO PREPARE

TOTAL TIME: 0 HUNDRED AND FIFTY-FIVE MINUTES

INGREDIENTS

1/2 c. honey

1/2 c. balsamic vinegar

1 tbsp. orange zest

tsp. chopped fresh oregano

medium yellow zucchini (about 1 lb.)

2 medium green zucchini (about 1 lb.)

salt, kosher

1 1/2 lb. Tyson Boneless Skinless Chicken Breasts, pounded to 1/2" thickness

extra-virgin olive oil

Black pepper, freshly ground

sea salt, such as Maldon

DIRECTIONS

In a small sauce pan over medium heat add honey and balsamic vinegar. Bring to a boil and simmer until slightly thickened, 10 minutes. Turn off heat; stir in orange zest and oregano. Reserve 1/4 cup for serving.

Meanwhile, trim off both ends of each zucchini. Using a mandoline or vegetable peeler, create long flat noodles by running the blade against the length of each zucchini. Season with salt and set aside.

Preheat grill on medium-high. Drizzle Tyson Boneless Skinless Chicken Breastswith olive oil and season with salt and pepper. Place chicken on grill and cook for 4 minutes on each side. Brush glaze onto chicken and cook until lightly charred all over and internal temperature reaches 170°, 2 to 3 minutes. Transfer to a clean plate and cover loosely with foil.

Bring an 8-quart stock pot of water to a boil and generously season with salt. Cook zucchini until al dente, 2 to 3 minutes, and drain. Slice chicken against the grain and serve over zucchini noodles with a drizzle of balsamic-honey glaze and a sprinkle of sea salt. Right away, serve. Parmesan-Crusted Salmon

4 SERVINGS YIELDS

PREP TIME: 0 HOURS 5 MINS

TIME TOTAL: ZERO HOURS AND TWENTY MINUTES

INGREDIENTS

1 c. grated Parmesan, plus more for garnish

1/4 c. chopped parsley, plus more for garnish

1 tblsp oregano (dried)

4 salmon pieces, about 2 lbs.

extra-virgin olive oil

salt, kosher

Black pepper, freshly ground

1 head broccoli, cut into florets

DIRECTIONS

In a small bowl combine parmesan, parsley and oregano. Rub salmon with olive oil and season with salt and black pepper. Place handful of cheese mixture on top of each piece; press down lightly to adhere.

Preheat oven to 425 degrees F. In a large cast iron skillet or nonstick pan over medium heat carefully place 2 pieces of salmon cheese-side down and sear until golden; about 2 to 3 minutes. Transfer to a plate cheese-side up. Wipe pan to remove excess cheese and repeat with remaining salmon. Place all salmon cheese-side up in the skillet and bake until cooked through, about 4 minutes.

Meanwhile, bring a large pot filled with salted water to a boil and cook broccoli for 2 minutes.

Plate salmon and drizzle with olive oil; garnish with parsley and parmesan. Serve immediately with broccoli. HEALTH BENEFITS OF PALEO DIET

Promotes healthy blood glucose

Improved insulin sensitivity

Lower blood pressure

Weight management including reduced waist circumference

Improved cholesterol balance

Improved satiety

Lower all-cause mortality

CONCLUSION

Our modern food is heavily processed, reliant on grains and sugars and modified fats. Most of the chronic health concerns that plague Americans today weren't as problematic in the past. The Paleo Diet posits that our food may be contributing to these diseases. As with any significant dietary change, it is best to consult your doctor before diving into the Paleo Diet. If you have the desire and time to prepare your own food and to get physically active, then a Paleolithic-type diet may work for you. Remember it is always important to work with your doctor and to pay attention to how your body responds.INGREDIENTS

6 slices bacon, cut into 1" pieces

1/2 onion, chopped

lb. Brussels sprouts, trimmed and quartered

salt, kosher

Black pepper, freshly ground

1/4 tsp. crushed red pepper flakes

garlic cloves, chopped

4 large eggs

DIRECTIONS

In a large skillet over medium heat, cook bacon until crispy. Turn off heat and transfer bacon to a paper towel-lined plate. Drain all but about 1 tablespoon bacon fat.

Turn heat back to medium and add onion and Brussels sprouts to the skillet. Cook, stirring occasionally, until vegetables begin to soften and turn golden. Season with salt, pepper, and red pepper flakes.

Add 2 tablespoons of water and cover skillet. Cook until Brussels sprouts are tender and water has evaporated, about 5 minutes. (If all the water evaporates before the Brussels sprouts are tender, add more water to skillet and cover for a couple minutes more.) Add garlic to skillet and cook until fragrant, 1 minute.

Using a wooden spoon, make four holes in the hash to reveal bottom of skillet. Crack an egg into each hole and season each egg with salt and pepper. Replace lid and cook until eggs are cooked to your liking, about 5 minutes for a just runny egg.

Sprinkle cooked bacon bits over entire skillet and serve warm

Grilled Chicken

4 SERVINGS YIELDS

TIME TO PREPARE: 15 MINUTES 0 HOUR

TIME TO COMPLETE: 0 HOURS 45 MINUTES TOTAL

INGREDIENTS

1/4 c. balsamic vinegar

3 tbsp.extra-virgin olive oil

tbsp. brown sugar

garlic cloves, chopped

1 tsp. dried thyme

1 tsp. dried rosemary

4 chicken breasts

salt, kosher

Black pepper, freshly ground

Freshly chopped parsley, for garnish

DIRECTIONS

In a medium bowl, whisk together balsamic vinegar, olive oil, brown sugar, garlic, and dried herbs, and season generously with salt and pepper. Reserve ¼ cup.

Add chicken to the bowl and toss to combine. Let marinate at least 20 minutes and up to overnight.

Preheat grill to medium high. Add chicken and grill, basting with reserved marinade, until cooked through, 6 minutes per side.

Before serving, top with parsley.

Paleo Chocolate Chip Cookies

YIELDS:

0 HOURS 10 MINUTES TO PREPARE

TOTAL TIME: 0 HOURS 25 MINS

INGREDIENTS

c. almond flour

1/2 tsp. baking soda

1/4 tsp. kosher salt

1/4 c. butter, room temperature

1/4 c. almond butter

honey (1 tbsp.)

1 large egg

1 tsp. pure vanilla extract

1 c. semisweet chocolate chips

Flaky sea salt

DIRECTIONS

Preheat oven to 350° and line a baking sheet with parchment paper. In a large bowl, whisk together almond flour, baking soda, and salt. Add butter, almond butter, honey, egg, and vanilla and, using a hand mixer, beat until combined.

Fold in chocolate chips until combined, then add tablespoonfuls of batter to prepared baking sheet. Sprinkle cookies with flaky sea salt.

Bake until edges are golden, 13 to 15 minutes.

Balsamic Grilled Chicken and Zucchini

SIZE OF YIELDS: 4 SIZE OF YIELDS: 4 SI

0 HOURS 10 MINUTES TO PREPARE

TOTAL TIME: 0 HUNDRED AND FIFTY-FIVE MINUTES

INGREDIENTS

1/2 c. honey

1/2 c. balsamic vinegar

1 tbsp. orange zest

tsp. chopped fresh oregano

medium yellow zucchini (about 1 lb.)

2 medium green zucchini (about 1 lb.)

salt, kosher

1 1/2 lb. Tyson Boneless Skinless Chicken Breasts, pounded to 1/2" thickness

extra-virgin olive oil

Black pepper, freshly ground

sea salt, such as Maldon

DIRECTIONS

In a small sauce pan over medium heat add honey and balsamic vinegar. Bring to a boil and simmer until slightly thickened, 10 minutes. Turn off heat; stir in orange zest and oregano. Reserve 1/4 cup for serving.

Meanwhile, trim off both ends of each zucchini. Using a mandoline or vegetable peeler, create long flat noodles by running the blade against the length of each zucchini. Season with salt and set aside.

Preheat grill on medium-high. Drizzle Tyson Boneless Skinless Chicken Breastswith olive oil and season with salt and pepper. Place chicken on grill and cook for 4 minutes on each side. Brush glaze onto chicken and cook until lightly charred all over and internal temperature reaches 170°, 2 to 3 minutes. Transfer to a clean plate and cover loosely with foil.

Bring an 8-quart stock pot of water to a boil and generously season with salt. Cook zucchini until al dente, 2 to 3 minutes, and drain. Slice chicken against the grain and serve over zucchini noodles with a drizzle of balsamic-honey glaze and a sprinkle of sea salt. Right away, serve. Parmesan-Crusted Salmon

4 SERVINGS YIELDS

PREP TIME: 0 HOURS 5 MINS

TIME TOTAL: ZERO HOURS AND TWENTY MINUTES

INGREDIENTS

1 c. grated Parmesan, plus more for garnish

1/4 c. chopped parsley, plus more for garnish

1 tblsp oregano (dried)

4 salmon pieces, about 2 lbs.

extra-virgin olive oil

salt, kosher

Black pepper, freshly ground

1 head broccoli, cut into florets

DIRECTIONS

In a small bowl combine parmesan, parsley and oregano. Rub salmon with olive oil and season

with salt and black pepper. Place handful of cheese mixture on top of each piece; press down lightly to adhere.

Preheat oven to 425 degrees F. In a large cast iron skillet or nonstick pan over medium heat carefully place 2 pieces of salmon cheese-side down and sear until golden; about 2 to 3 minutes. Transfer to a plate cheese-side up. Wipe pan to remove excess cheese and repeat with remaining salmon.

Place all salmon cheese-side up in the skillet and bake until cooked through, about 4 minutes.

Meanwhile, bring a large pot filled with salted water to a boil and cook broccoli for 2 minutes.

Plate salmon and drizzle with olive oil; garnish with parsley and parmesan. Serve immediately with broccoli. HEALTH BENEFITS OF PALEO DIET

Promotes healthy blood glucose

Improved insulin sensitivity

Lower blood pressure

Weight management including reduced waist circumference

Improved cholesterol balance

Improved satiety

Lower all-cause mortality

Chapter Five

CONCLUSION

Our modern food is heavily processed, reliant on grains and sugars and modified fats. Most of the chronic health concerns that plague Americans today weren't as problematic in the past. The Paleo Diet posits that our food may be contributing to these diseases. As with any significant dietary change, it is best to consult your doctor before diving into the Paleo Diet. If you have the desire and time to prepare your own food and to get physically active, then a Paleolithic-type diet may work for you. Remember it is always important to work with your doctor and to pay attention to how your body responds.